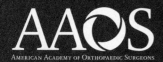

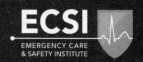

CPR and AED

Meets CPR and ECC Guidelines

EIGHTH EDITION

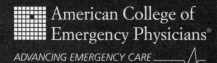
American College of
Emergency Physicians®
ADVANCING EMERGENCY CARE

Authors

Alton L. Thygerson, EdD, FAWM

Steven M. Thygerson, PhD, MSPH, CIH

Justin S. Thygerson, PhD, CSP

Medical Editors

Alfonso Mejia, MD, MPH, FAAOS

Ira Nemeth, MD, FACEP, FAEMS

Bob Elling, MPA, EMT-P

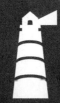

JONES & BARTLETT
LEARNING

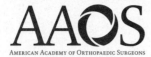

AMERICAN ACADEMY OF ORTHOPAEDIC SURGEONS

World Headquarters
Jones & Bartlett Learning
5 Wall Street
Burlington, MA 01803
978-443-5000
info@jblearning.com
www.psglearning.com

Library of Congress Cataloging-in-Publication Data
Library of Congress Cataloging-in-Publication Data unavailable at time of printing.

LCCN: 2021910430

978-1-284-23564-7

6048

Printed in the United States of America
25 24   10 9 8 7 6 5 4 3

Brief Contents

Contents

Skill Sheets

Welcome

Welcome to the Emergency Care and Safety Institute

Welcome to the Emergency Care and Safety Institute (ECSI), brought to you by the American Academy of Orthopaedic Surgeons (AAOS) and the American College of Emergency Physicians (ACEP).

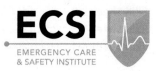

ECSI is an internationally renowned organization that provides training and certifications that meet job-related requirements as defined by regulatory authorities such as the Occupational Safety and Health Administration (OSHA), the Joint Commission, and State offices of Emergency Medical Services (EMS), Education, Transportation, and Health. Our courses are delivered throughout a range of industries and markets worldwide, including colleges and universities, business and industry, governments, public safety agencies, hospitals, private training companies, and secondary school systems.

ECSI programs are offered in association with the AAOS and ACEP. AAOS, the world's largest medical association of musculoskeletal specialists, is known as the original name in EMS publishing, putting out the first EMS textbook ever in 1971, and ACEP is widely recognized as the leading name in all of emergency medicine.

ECSI Course Catalog

Individuals seeking training from ECSI can choose from among various traditional classroom-based courses or alternative online courses, such as:

- Advanced Cardiac Life Support (ACLS)
- Basic Life Support (BLS) for Health Care Providers
- Bloodborne and Airborne Pathogens
- CPR and AED
- First Aid (standard, advanced, pediatric, pet, sports, wilderness)

ECSI offers a wide range of textbooks, instructor and student support materials, and interactive technology, including online courses. ECSI student manuals are the center of an integrated teaching and learning system that offers resources to better support instructors and train students. The instructor supplements provide practical, hands-on, time-saving tools such as slides in PowerPoint format, skills demonstration videos, and web-based distance learning resources. Technology resources provide interactive exercises and simulations to help students become prepared for any emergency.

Documents attesting to ECSI's recognitions of satisfactory course completion will be issued to those who successfully meet the course requirements. Written acknowledgment of a participant's successful course completion is provided in the form of a Course Completion Card, issued by the ECSI.

Visit www.ECSInstitute.org today!

Preface

2020 Guideline Updates and the COVID-19 Pandemic

This book exceeds the requirements of the 2020 American Heart Association (AHA) Emergency Cardiovascular Care (ECC) Guidelines and the 2020 International Liaison Committee on Resuscitation (ILCOR) Consensus on Science with Treatment Recommendations (CoSTR). At this time, we find ourselves in the middle of a 100-year event: the COVID-19 pandemic. These updates were made with the pandemic in mind.

Although we are perhaps more mindful than ever of the importance of personal protective equipment (PPE) during treatment, readers will still notice some variability throughout this textbook with regard to PPE worn by layperson responders as they care for those who are injured or ill. They may also question the inclusion of skills and techniques that are discouraged in the context of COVID-19.

We have tried, throughout the text, to apply the best current knowledge and practices available. However, that science is developing rapidly, and we will make every attempt to make supplemental material available that reflects the most updated knowledge.

Face Masks

Prior to 2020, the level of PPE commonly worn by all layperson responders while providing treatment typically included disposable gloves when possible. Face masks are now standard equipment for all interpersonal encounters, not just during treatment. Social distancing guidelines mandate the use of masks in public. People without symptoms can still be infected with the virus and thus transmit it to others. Asking everyone to wear a mask during treatment can make those encounters safer.

Art and Photos

Revising the illustrations and images throughout the book has been a challenge. Organizing photo shoots has been dramatically hindered by necessary social distancing restrictions. For this reason, we ensured that layperson responders and other relevant parties were wearing face masks and appropriate eye protection in any new images that were shot for this textbook. However, we were not able to update all the photos to reflect new practice guidelines. It is certainly our hope that by the time the next edition is published, our knowledge of best practices with regard to PPE will be more static and there will be more consistency in the appearance of PPE in images throughout the book.

Cardiopulmonary Resuscitation

This revised book includes coverage of mouth-to-mouth cardiopulmonary resuscitation (CPR) and mouth-to-barrier CPR. These techniques are still key competencies for the layperson responder whose partner or family member has, for example, had a sudden cardiac arrest. This book also includes coverage of hands-only CPR for instances where the layperson responder is unable or unwilling to provide rescue breaths. During the COVID-19 pandemic, ILCOR recommends that layperson responders consider hands-only CPR and defibrillation for treating those who are not members of the responder's household and consider rescue breaths and chest compressions for infants and children.

Acknowledgments

The authors, the medical editors, the Jones & Bartlett Learning Public Safety Group, the American Academy of Orthopaedic Surgeons (AAOS), and the American College of Emergency Physicians (ACEP) would like to thank all of the reviewers who generously offered their time, expertise, and talent to the making of this eighth edition.

Reviewers

Ken Bartz, AEMT
EMS Instructor Coordinator
Southwest Wisconsin Technical College
Fennimore, Wisconsin

Kent Courtney
Paramedic, Firefighter, Rescue Technician, Educator
Essential Safety Training and Consulting
Lake Montezuma, Arizona

Chance Cummings
Lieutenant, Paramedic, EMS Liaison Officer
Starkville Fire Department
Starkville, Mississippi

James W. Fogal, NRP, MA
Auburn University
Auburn, Alabama

Fidel O. Garcia
Paramedic
Professional EMS Education
Grand Junction, Colorado

Michele M. Hoffman, MS, Ed, RN, NREMT
James City County Fire Department
Williamsburg, Virginia

Benjamin McKenna, MA
AHA CTC Coordinator
University of South Alabama
Mobile, Alabama

Gregory S. Neiman, MS, NRP, NCEE
EMS Liaison
Virginia Commonwealth University Health
Richmond, Virginia

William H. Turner, MS, NRP, EMSI
Assistant Professor, Director of Emergency Medical Technology
Shawnee State University
Portsmouth, Ohio

Josh Weiner, NRP, FP-C
Minneapolis, Minnesota

Raymond C. Whatley Jr., MBA, NRP, CEM
Emergency Health Services Program
George Washington University
Washington, District of Columbia

Christopher C. Williams, PhD, NRP
Guilford County EMS
Greensboro, North Carolina

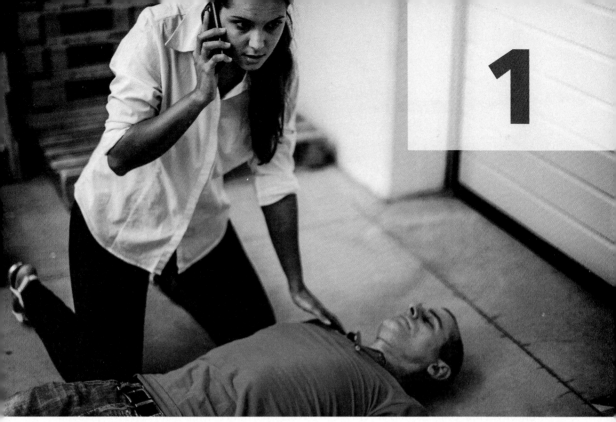

© pixelaway/Shutterstock.

Introduction

Introduction

More than 300,000 cardiac arrests occur annually in the United States. Approximately 10% of affected individuals survive, as reported by the Centers for Disease Control and Prevention. The aim of this manual is to help increase that percentage. If more people learn how to administer cardiopulmonary resuscitation (CPR), the survival percentage will increase.

Cardio refers to the heart and *pulmonary* refers to the lungs. CPR consists of moving blood to the heart and brain by giving chest compressions and providing rescue breaths to place oxygen into the person's lungs. Proper and prompt CPR serves as a holding action until defibrillation and advanced care can be provided.

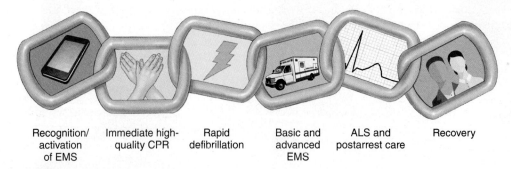

| Recognition/ activation of EMS | Immediate high- quality CPR | Rapid defibrillation | Basic and advanced EMS | ALS and postarrest care | Recovery |

FIGURE 1-1 Out-of-hospital chain of survival.
Abbreviation: ALS = advanced life support.
Reprinted with permission ©2020 American Heart Association, Inc.

One way of describing the ideal sequence of care that should take place when a cardiac arrest occurs is to compare it to the links in a chain. Each link is dependent on the others for strength and success. In this way, the links form a chain of survival. The six events (links) that must occur rapidly and in an integrated manner during cardiac arrest outside of a hospital are as follows (**FIGURE 1-1**):

1. *Recognition and action.* Responders must recognize the early warning signs of cardiac arrest and immediately call 9-1-1 to activate emergency medical services (EMS).
2. *CPR.* The chest compressions delivered during CPR circulate blood to the heart and brain. Effective chest compressions are critical to buying time until a defibrillator and EMS personnel are available.
3. *Defibrillation.* Administering a shock to the heart can restore the heartbeat in some people. Time is a critical factor. The earlier the shock, the better the chance of success.
4. *Advanced care.* Paramedics provide advanced cardiac life support to people experiencing sudden cardiac arrest. This support includes providing intravenous fluids, medications, advanced airway devices, and rapid transport to the hospital.
5. *Postarrest care.* The hospital can provide lifesaving medications, surgical procedures, and advanced medical care to enable the person experiencing sudden cardiac arrest to survive and recover.
6. *Recovery.* Identifies the system of care to support recovery and plan treatment and rehabilitation for cardiac arrest survivors as they transition from the hospital to home and return to their daily activities.

Willingness to Help

At some time, everyone will have to decide whether or not to help another person. Unless the decision to act in an emergency is considered well in advance of an actual emergency, the many obstacles that make it difficult or unpleasant for you to help are almost certain to impede action. One important strategy that people use to avoid action is to refuse (consciously or unconsciously) to acknowledge the emergency. Many emergencies do not look like the ones portrayed on television, and the uncertainty of an actual emergency can make it easier for people to avoid acknowledging the emergency.

People are more likely to promptly get involved at the time of an emergency if they have previously considered the possibility of helping others. Thus, the most important time to make the decision to help is before ever encountering an emergency. Deciding to help is an attitude about emergencies and about one's ability to deal with emergencies. It is an attitude that takes time to develop and is affected by a number of factors. To develop such a helping attitude, people must do the following:

- Understand the importance of helping a person.
- Feel confident about helping someone, even if someone else is present.
- Be willing to take the time to help.
- Be able to put the potential risks of helping in perspective.
- Feel comfortable about taking charge, if needed, at an emergency scene. This is accomplished with ongoing competency in the skill drills in your training as well as experience, either actual or simulated.
- Feel comfortable about seeing a person who is bleeding or who appears dead.

A bystander could always find excuses for not helping in emergency situations. It is up to you to decide to help before an emergency occurs.

Standard of Care

The level of care required of a lay responder is referred to as the *standard of care*. A lay responder cannot provide the same level of care as a physician or an emergency medical technician. When you are providing CPR, you must do the following to meet the standard of care: (1) do what is expected of someone with first aid training and experience, working under similar conditions, and (2) treat the person to the best of your ability.

Actions to Take Before Helping

After recognizing an emergency and deciding to help, do the following:

1. *Size up the scene.*
   - Are there any dangerous hazards present?
   - How many people are in need of first aid?
   - What could be wrong with the person(s)?
   - What happened?
   - Are bystanders available to help?
2. *Assume you have consent (permission) to help an unresponsive person.*
3. *Call for professional medical care if it is needed.* If you are in a commercial building, another option is to contact the building's emergency response team or security staff. If you have a mobile phone, it may be possible to call for professional medical care and attend to the person at the same time.
4. *Prevent disease transmission.* Avoid contact with blood and other body fluids by putting on personal protective equipment (PPE), if available. PPE includes disposable medical exam gloves, breathing masks with a one-way valve, and face shields.

   Note: Every situation is different. Depending on your relationship with the injured person (eg, spouse, child), you may not need to wear PPE if you know their health history.

Scene Size-up

You should perform a scene size-up every time you respond to an emergency. As you approach the scene, ask yourself a series of questions as shown in **FLOWCHART 1-1**.

Flowchart 1-1 Scene Size-up

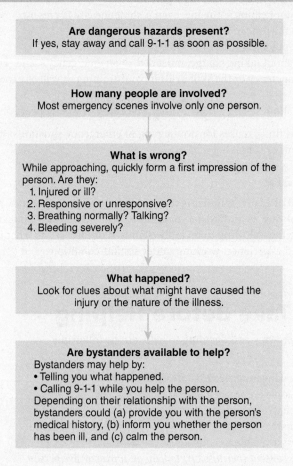

Are dangerous hazards present?
If yes, stay away and call 9-1-1 as soon as possible.

How many people are involved?
Most emergency scenes involve only one person.

What is wrong?
While approaching, quickly form a first impression of the person. Are they:
1. Injured or ill?
2. Responsive or unresponsive?
3. Breathing normally? Talking?
4. Bleeding severely?

What happened?
Look for clues about what might have caused the injury or the nature of the illness.

Are bystanders available to help?
Bystanders may help by:
• Telling you what happened.
• Calling 9-1-1 while you help the person.
Depending on their relationship with the person, bystanders could (a) provide you with the person's medical history, (b) inform you whether the person has been ill, and (c) calm the person.

Seeking Professional Medical Care

You should recognize when professional medical care is needed and know how to get it. This includes learning how and when to access EMS by calling 9-1-1 and how to activate the on-site emergency response system (**FIGURE 1-2**).

How to Call for Professional Medical Care

When calling 9-1-1, be sure to speak slowly and clearly. Be ready to give the dispatcher the following information:

- The person's location
- The phone number you are calling from and your name

- A brief account of what happened
- The number of people needing help and any special conditions at the scene
- A description of the person's condition and what is being done

Listen to what the dispatcher tells you to do. If possible, keep the phone at the side of the person needing help. Do not hang up until the dispatcher tells you to.

9-1-1 Service

According to the National Emergency Number Association and the Canadian Radio-television and Tele-communications Commission, about 97% of the populations of the United States and Canada are covered by some type of 9-1-1 service. Many areas also have Enhanced 9-1-1, which lets the dispatcher see the caller's phone number and address if the call is placed from a landline. When you call 9-1-1 from a mobile phone, Enhanced 9-1-1 cannot identify your exact address, because mobile phone signals only provide a general location. Because of this key difference, make sure that you know your exact address or location to give to the 9-1-1 dispatcher.

Legal Aspects of Helping

Although you may not be legally required to help another person, most people believe helping others is the right thing to do. You must help when you have a legal duty to act (**FIGURE 1-3**):

- Employment requires it (eg, job description)
- Preexisting relationship exists (eg, parent-child, teacher-student, driver-passenger)

Confidential Information

Lay responders might learn confidential information. It is important that you be extremely cautious about revealing information that you learn while caring for someone. The law recognizes that people have the right to privacy. Do not discuss what you know with anyone other than those who have a medical need

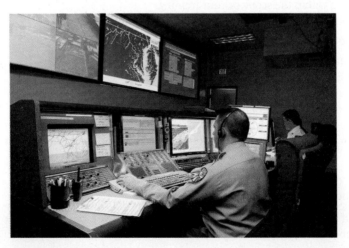

FIGURE 1-2 9-1-1 dispatch center.
© Jones & Bartlett Learning. Courtesy of MIEMSS.

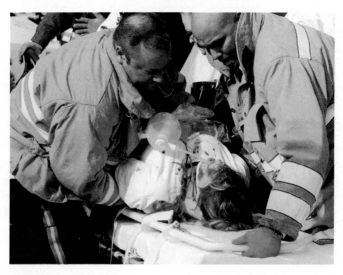

FIGURE 1-3 You must help a person when you have a legal duty to do so.
© Spiritartist/iStock photo.

to know. The exception to this rule is when state laws require the reporting of certain incidents, such as rape, abuse, and gunshot wounds.

Good Samaritan Laws

Good Samaritan laws provide reasonable protection against lawsuits and encourage people to help others during an emergency. Laws are different from state to state but in general, the following conditions must be met:

- You are acting with good intentions.
- You are providing care without expectation of compensation.
- You are acting within the scope of your training.
- You are not acting in a grossly negligent (reckless) manner.

Negligent actions include:

- Giving substandard care
- Withholding care when you have a legal duty to act
- Causing injury or harm
- Attempting to provide care that exceeds your level of training
- Abandoning the person (starting care and then stopping or leaving without ensuring that a rescuer with the same or a higher level of training will continue to care for the person)

Consent

Types of consent include:

- Informed: If a person who is choking is responsive, ask if you can help. You do not need to ask if you can help if the person is unresponsive.
- Implied: Assume consent for an unresponsive person.
- For children: If a parent or legal guardian is unavailable, implied consent can be assumed.

Preventing Disease Transmission

Body fluids (such as blood, saliva, and stool) can sometimes carry disease-producing germs. Appropriate PPE should always be worn. In cases where gloves are not available, put your hands in plastic bags. Be sure to wash your hands thoroughly after administering aid, even if gloves are worn. If soap and water are unavailable, use an alcohol-based hand cleaner. Also wash or rinse any exposed areas including eyes, nose, or mouth. Inform your supervisor if you are at work and be sure to contact your primary care physician if you are exposed to body fluids. Take proper precautions to protect against diseases such as:

- HIV/AIDS
- Hepatitis B virus
- Hepatitis C virus
- Tuberculosis
- Meningitis
- COVID-19

Personal Protective Equipment

Avoid contact with blood and other body fluids by putting on PPE, which includes:

- Disposable medical exam gloves (use latex-free gloves, if possible; nitrile gloves are recommended, **FIGURE 1-4**)
- Eye protection (face shield)
- Mouth-to-barrier device (pocket mask or face shield, **FIGURE 1-5**)
- Face covering (face mask or face shield) to prevent disease transmission (**FIGURE 1-6**)

Note: For years, the term *pocket mask* has referred to a mouth-to-barrier device used when giving rescue breaths during CPR (see Figure 1-5A). CPR pocket masks are very different compared with face masks worn in public for disease prevention (such as those used during the COVID-19 pandemic; see Figure 1-6A). The term *face shield* can apply to two different pieces of equipment: those for CPR (see Figure 1-5B) and those for public health (see Figure 1-6B).

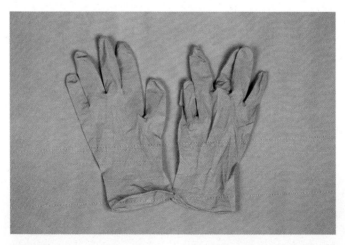

FIGURE 1-4 Disposable gloves.
© Jones & Bartlett Learning. Photographed by Kimberly Potvin.

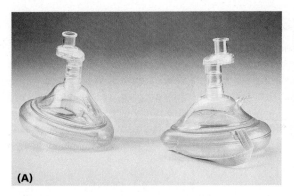

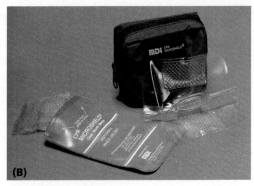

FIGURE 1-5 Mouth-to-barrier devices. **A.** Pocket mask for CPR. **B.** Face shields for CPR.
© Jones & Bartlett Learning. Courtesy of MIEMSS.

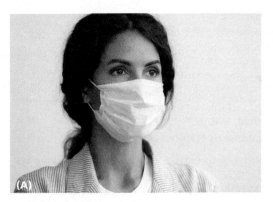

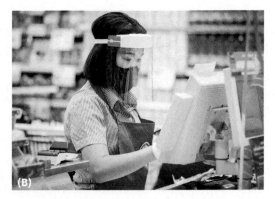

FIGURE 1-6 A. Face mask for public health. **B.** Face shield for public health.
A. © fizkes/Shutterstock; B. © pixfly/Shutterstock.

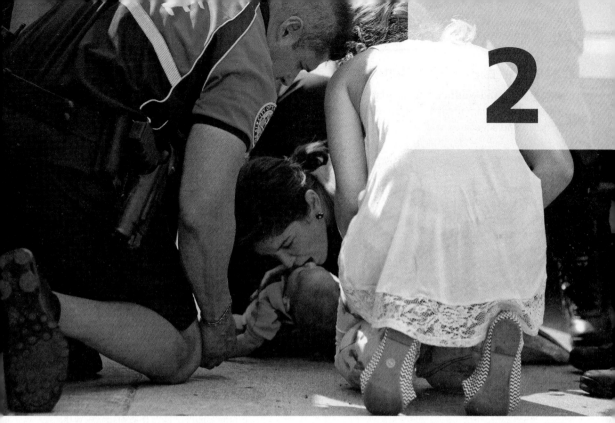

© Al Díaz/Miami Herald/AP Photo.

Cardiopulmonary Resuscitation

Heart Attack and Cardiac Arrest

The meaning of these two terms—*heart attack* and *cardiac arrest*—confuses many people.

A heart attack happens when the blood supply to the heart muscle is suddenly reduced or blocked. If the blocked artery is not reopened quickly, the affected part of the heart begins to die. The longer a person goes without treatment, the greater the damage and can lead to a cardiac arrest.

A cardiac arrest happens when the heart stops beating or when a rapid irregular rhythm (ventricular fibrillation) suddenly develops. It is one of the leading causes of death.

Care for a Person Having a Heart Attack

Heart attacks can be difficult to determine, so it is important to know the signs and symptoms as well as the most appropriate medical facility to transport these patients. This will help you be prepared to provide quick and accurate care.

What to Look For	What to Do

Though sometimes difficult to determine, symptoms of a heart attack can include:
 	
■ Chest discomfort that feels like pressure, squeezing, or fullness, usually in the center of the chest. It may also be felt in the jaw, shoulder, arms, or back.
 	
■ Sweating
 	
■ Lightheadedness or dizziness
 	
■ Nausea or vomiting
 	
■ Numbness, aching, or tingling in an arm (most often the left arm)
 	
■ Shortness of breath
 	
■ Weakness or fatigue, especially in older adults
 	
Women and the elderly experience the typical signs and symptoms of a heart attack. However, they are more likely than men to have milder signs and symptoms of a heart attack that can extend over many hours, days, or weeks leading up to the heart attack, such as:
 	
■ Shortness of breath
 	
■ Nausea or vomiting
 	
■ An ache in the chest
 	
■ Sore jaw
 	
■ Strange feeling in arm
 	
■ Upper back pain
 	
■ Flulike symptoms
 	
■ Dizziness
	1. Have the person sit, with knees raised, and lean against a stable but comfortable support (eg, wall, tree trunk, fence post). Try to keep the person calm. **DO NOT** allow the person to walk. Doing so can put more stress on the heart.
	
	2. Call 9-1-1 immediately. **DO NOT** drive the person to a medical facility; wait for EMS to arrive.
	
	3. While waiting for EMS to arrive:
	   • Loosen any tight clothing.
	   • Ask if the person takes any chest pain medication (eg, nitroglycerin) for a known heart condition, and if so, help them take it.
	   • If the person is alert, able to swallow, not allergic to aspirin, and has no signs of a stroke, help the person take one adult aspirin (325 mg) or two to four low-dose aspirins (81 mg each). Pulverize or crush the aspirin or have the person chew the aspirin before swallowing for faster results.
	   • Monitor breathing. If the person becomes unresponsive and stops breathing, begin CPR. If they are unresponsive and are breathing, place them on their side in the recovery position. (See page 21.)

Care for a Person Experiencing Cardiac Arrest

When a person's heart stops beating, they need to quickly receive CPR, defibrillation, and the help of emergency medical service (EMS) professionals.

Cardiopulmonary resuscitation (CPR) consists of using chest compressions and rescue breaths to maintain circulatory blood flow and oxygenation during cardiac arrest. Some people worry about hurting the person (eg, breaking ribs), but that is unlikely. Moreover, any harm done is less of a problem than having a nonfunctioning heart.

CPR for a child is identical to that given for an adult with a few key differences.

An automated external defibrillator (AED) is an electronic device that analyzes the heart rhythm and if necessary prompts the rescuer to deliver an electric shock, known as defibrillation, to the heart of a person in cardiac arrest.

Cardiopulmonary Resuscitation

For a life-threatening condition (cardiac arrest), doing something is always better than doing nothing! This is not only the case for the person suffering, but also for your benefit as the first aid responder. Even if unsuccessful, you will know that you tried everything you could to save the person's life.

Adult or Child CPR

Before helping, take the appropriate actions. When you see a motionless adult or child, scan the scene for hazards that could endanger your life. Being injured yourself could prevent you from providing CPR.

If there is massive extremity hemorrhaging, quickly apply or have someone else apply a tourniquet.

Use the **RAB-CAB** mnemonic to remember the sequence of what to do when providing adult or child CPR. RAB-CAB stands for:

R = Responsive?
A = Activate EMS and obtain an AED
B = Breathing?
C = Compressions
A = Airway
B = Breaths

R = Responsive?

Tap the person's shoulder and shout, "Are you okay?" to decide if the person is responsive or unresponsive.

If...	Then...
The person is responsive (eg, speaks, moves)	• Ask if you can help them. • If they agree, use the **SAMPLE** mnemonic (symptoms; allergies; medications; pertinent past medical history; last oral intake; events leading up to the injury or illness) questions to obtain relevant medical information. • If they appear to have been injured, look for and ask about **DOTS** (deformities; open wounds; tenderness; swelling). • Provide care for what is found and if necessary, call 9-1-1.
The person is unresponsive (eg, does not answer, move, or moan)	• Continue to the next step, *A = Activate*

A = Activate EMS and Obtain an AED

Shout for nearby help.

If...	Then...
Someone comes to help	• Have them activate EMS by calling 9-1-1 or local emergency number and obtain an AED while you continue providing care. • If a mobile phone is used, put it on speaker mode and place it at the person's side, if possible, to hear the dispatcher's directions.

If...	Then...
You are alone and the person is an adult	- Call 9-1-1 and obtain an AED. - If a phone is not available, leave the person to call 9-1-1 and obtain an AED. After making the call, return and continue providing care.
The person is a child (between age 1 and puberty)	- If you are alone, give 5 sets of compressions and 2 breaths before calling 9-1-1. - If someone arrives to help, have them call 9-1-1 and obtain an AED while you continue giving CPR.

B = Breathing?

Observe the person from neck to waist for movement (rise and fall); take 5 to 10 seconds.

If...	Then...
The person is unresponsive and breathing normally	- Place the person on their side in the recovery position to keep the airway open. (See page 21.) - Stay with the person and monitor their breathing until EMS arrives.
The person is unresponsive and not breathing or is only gasping (may sound like a quick inhalation or like a groan or snore)	- Place the person face up on a flat, firm surface. - Continue to the next step, C = Compressions

C = Compressions

Give chest compressions.

1. Remove enough clothing to locate the correct hand position for compressions and to apply an AED when it arrives on the scene.
2. For an adult, place the heel of one hand on the center of the person's chest and on the lower half of their breastbone (sternum).
3. Place your other hand on top of the first one with your fingers interlocked. Hold your fingers off the person's chest and point them directly away from you. **DO NOT** cross your hands. For a child, use one hand; however, depending upon the child's size and your size, using two hands may be necessary.
4. Keep your arms straight and elbows locked, with your shoulders positioned directly over your hands.
5. Push hard and straight down on the breastbone (sternum), at least 2 inches (5 cm) for an adult and about 2 inches or one-third the depth of the chest for a child. Use your upper body's weight to compress the chest. **DO NOT** rock back and forth.
6. Push fast: Give 30 compressions (100 to 120 compressions per minute). To maintain the compression rate, follow the beats of the Bee Gees song "Stayin' Alive", the beats from a CPR smartphone app that was previously installed and is quickly accessible, or a dispatcher's directions heard over a mobile phone speaker.
7. Push smoothly: **DO NOT** bounce or jab and **DO NOT** stop at the top or bottom of a compression.
8. Allow the chest to fully recoil after each compression. **DO NOT** lean on the chest.

A = Airway

Open the person's airway using the head tilt–chin lift maneuver *only* when a spinal neck (cervical vertebrae) injury is *not* suspected. When a spinal neck injury *is* suspected, first aid responders should not use immobilization devices (eg, cervical collars) and, instead, should restrict spinal motion (eg, placing their hands on the sides of the person's head to hold it still):

1. Take your hand nearest the person's head and place it on their forehead; apply pressure to tilt the head back.
2. Place two fingers of your other hand under the bony part of the person's jaw (near the chin) and lift. Avoid pressing on the soft tissues under the jaw.
3. Tilt the head backward.

B = Breaths

Give 2 breaths:

1. Pinch the person's nose shut and make a tight seal with your mouth on the mouth-to-barrier device or the person's mouth. When possible, use a mouth-to-barrier device to prevent potential disease transmission. If unwilling or unable to give breaths (ie, seriously injured mouth, ineffective seal, mouth cannot be opened), give compression-only CPR. (See page 20.)
2. Give 2 breaths, each lasting 1 second (take a normal breath for yourself after each breath). **DO NOT** blow too forcefully or for too long.
3. Watch for chest rise to determine if your breaths go in.
4. Allow for chest deflation after each breath.
5. Follow the actions in the table.

If...	Then...
You see the chest rise after giving 2 breaths	Give sets of 30 chest compressions followed by 2 breaths.
The first breath does not cause the chest to rise	Retilt the person's head and give a second breath.
Retilting the head and the second breath still does not make the chest rise	• An object may be blocking the person's airway. • Give CPR with one change: after each set of 30 compressions and before giving breaths, open the mouth, look for an object in the back of the throat, and if seen, remove it. **DO NOT** use blind finger sweeps in those with a foreign-body airway obstruction.
You cannot use the person's mouth (eg, seriously injured mouth, ineffective seal, mouth cannot be opened, person is in water)	• Use the head tilt–chin lift maneuver. • Seal your mouth around the person's nose and provide breaths. Use a barrier device when possible. • Alternately, use compression-only CPR. (See page 20.)
The person vomits or there is fluid in the mouth	Roll the person onto their side and clear the mouth using a gloved finger or piece of gauze. Then, roll the person onto their back and continue care.

Continue sets of 30 chest compressions and 2 breaths until:

- An AED arrives (follow the manufacturer's directions for pad placement). After the AED pads are placed on the exposed chest, the AED will advise if CPR should be continued.

- The person begins breathing.
- Other rescuer(s) (eg, EMS personnel, trained layperson) replace you and gives CPR.
- The scene becomes unsafe. The person should be moved to a nearby safer location before continuing CPR.
- You are alone and become physically exhausted and unable to continue.

If another person is present, they could help by giving chest compressions while you give breaths, or vice versa. If the other person is not trained in CPR, you can coach them on how to perform chest compressions and how to give breaths. Switching places after every 5 sets (about every 2 minutes) helps avoid fatigue. The concern about contracting a disease from giving breaths can be remedied by: (1) giving compression-only CPR or (2) having both rescuers using their own mouth-to-barrier device while giving breaths.

Refer to **SKILL SHEET 2-1** for the steps and techniques for adult or child CPR.

Skill Sheet 2-1 Adult and Child CPR

Note: Whenever possible, use a mouth-to-barrier device to prevent disease transmission. Use the **RAB-CAB** mnemonic to remember what to do.

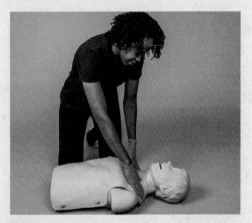 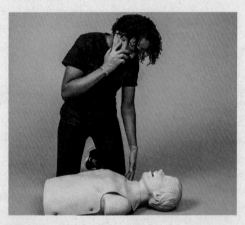

1 **R = Responsive?**
Tap the person's shoulder and shout, "Are you okay?"
- a. If the person responds, ask SAMPLE history questions and look for and ask about DOTS.
- b. If the person does not respond, continue to the next step, *A = Activate.*

2 **A = Activate EMS and obtain an AED.**
- a. Shout for nearby help.
- b. If someone responds, have them call 9-1-1 and obtain an AED while you provide care.
- c. If no one comes and you are alone with an adult, call 9-1-1 and put the phone on speaker mode so that you can prepare to follow the dispatcher's instructions. If a phone is not available, leave the person to locate a phone and obtain an AED.
- d. If no one comes and you are alone with a child, give 5 sets of 30 chest compressions and 2 breaths before calling 9-1-1.

Skill Sheet 2-1 Adult and Child CPR *(Continued)*

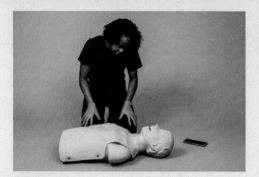

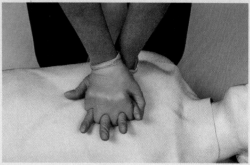

3 **B = Breathing?**
   a. Place the person face up on a flat, firm surface.
   b. Take 5 to 10 seconds to observe the person from the neck to waist for movement (rise and fall).
   c. If the person is not breathing or is only gasping, continue to the next step, *C = Compressions*.

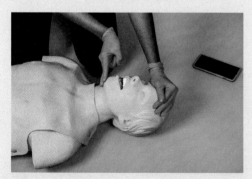

5 **A = Airway.**
Open the person's airway:
   a. Take your hand that is nearest to the person's head and place it on their forehead; apply pressure to tilt the head back.
   b. Place two fingers of your other hand under the bony part of the person's jaw (near the chin) and lift. Avoid pressing on soft tissues under the jaw.
   c. Tilt the head backward.

4 **C = Compressions.**
Provide chest compressions:
   a. Move enough clothing to locate the correct hand position for compressions and where to apply an AED when it arrives on the scene.
   b. For an adult:
      • Place the heel of one hand on the center of the person's chest and on the lower half of their breastbone (sternum).
      • Place your other hand on top of the first one with your fingers interlocked. Hold your fingers off the person's chest and point them directly away from you; **DO NOT** cross your hands.
   c. For a child:
      • Use one hand; however, depending upon the child's size and your size, using two hands may be necessary.
   d. Keep your arms straight and elbows locked, with your shoulders positioned directly over your hands.
   e. Push hard and straight down on the breastbone (sternum), at least 2 inches (5 cm) for an adult and about 2 inches (5 cm) or one-third the depth of the chest for a child. Use your upper body's weight to compress the chest. **DO NOT** rock back and forth.
   f. Push fast: 100 to 120 compressions per minute. It may be easier to push to the beat to the Bee Gees song "Stayin' Alive" or the beat from a CPR smartphone app that was previously installed and is quickly accessible.
   g. Push smoothly: **DO NOT** bounce or jab and **DO NOT** stop at the top or bottom of a compression.
   h. Allow the chest to fully recoil after each compression. **DO NOT** lean on the chest.

(Continues)

Skill Sheet 2-1 Adult and Child CPR   *(Continued)*

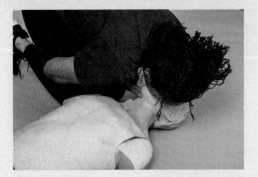

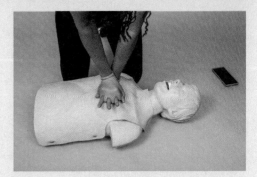

6 **B = Breaths.**
Give 2 breaths, using a mouth-to-barrier device when possible:
   a. Pinch the person's nose shut and make a tight seal with your mouth on the mouth-to-barrier device or the person's mouth. If unwilling or unable to give breaths, give compression-only CPR instead.
   b. Give 2 breaths, each lasting 1 second. **DO NOT** blow too forcefully or for too long. (Take a normal breath for yourself after each breath.)
   c. Watch for chest rise to determine if your breaths go in.
   d. Allow for chest deflation after each breath.
   e. If you see chest rise after the 2 breaths, give 30 chest compressions.
   f. If the first breath does not make the chest rise, retilt the person's head and give a second breath. If the second breath does not make the chest rise, begin CPR (30 compressions and 2 breaths). Each time before giving the first of the 2 breaths, open the mouth and look for an object; if seen, remove it.

7 Continue sets of 30 compressions and 2 breaths until one of the following occurs:
   • The person begins breathing.
   • EMS arrives and takes over.
   • You become physically exhausted and are unable to continue.
If a bystander is present, they could help by giving chest compressions while you perform rescue breathing, or vice versa.

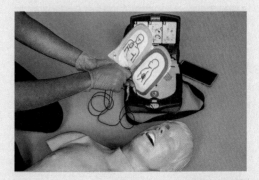

8 When an AED becomes available, use it as soon as possible. Follow the manufacturer's directions for pad placement. (See Chapter 4, *Automated External Defibrillation*.)

Infant CPR

To perform CPR on an infant, follow the steps in **SKILL SHEET 2-2**.

Skill Sheet 2-2 Infant CPR

Note: Use the **RAB-CAB** mnemonic to remember what to do.

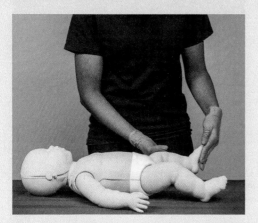

1 **R = Responsive?**
Tap the bottom of the infant's foot and shout their name.
  a. If the infant moves, cries, or reacts, they are responsive. Continue first aid.
  b. If the infant does not move, cry, or react, they are unresponsive. Continue to the next step, *A = Activate*.

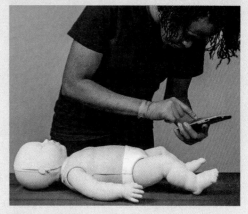

2 **A = Activate EMS and obtain an AED.**
  a. Shout for nearby help.
  b. If someone responds, have them call 9-1-1, set the phone to speaker mode, and obtain an AED while you start CPR. If a phone is not available, have them leave to call 9-1-1 and obtain an AED while you start CPR.
  c. If you are alone, call 9-1-1, set the phone on speaker mode, and perform CPR (30 chest compressions and 2 breaths for 5 cycles), and then obtain an AED. If you are alone without a phone, perform CPR for 5 cycles and then obtain an AED.

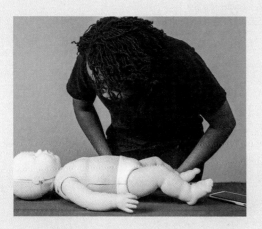

3 **B = Breathing?**
Take 5 to 10 seconds to check for breathing or only gasping by observing the infant's face and chest movement. If the infant is not breathing or only gasping, continue to the next step, *C = Compressions*.

(Continues)

Skill Sheet 2-2 Infant CPR *(Continued)*

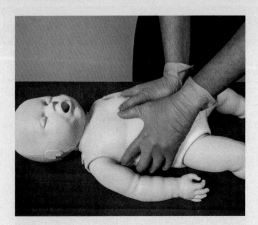 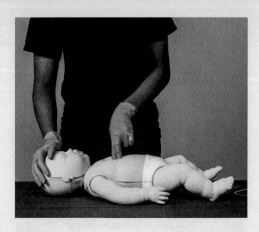

4 **C = Compressions.**

Place the infant face up on a flat, firm surface. If possible, use an elevated surface (eg, table, cabinet top). Single rescuers can use either the encircling thumbs technique or the two-finger technique. If the rescuer cannot physically encircle the infant's chest, use the two-finger technique.

4a. *Encircling Thumbs Technique (left photo):*
  a. Place both thumbs on the lower third of the breastbone (sternum), both touching the imaginary nipple line and the fingers encircling around the infant's back and chest.
  b. Give 30 chest compressions:
    • Push hard: about 1.5 inches (4 cm) straight down.
    • Push fast: to the beat of the Bee Gees song "Stayin' Alive".
    • At the end of each compression, let the infant's chest come back up to its normal position.

4b. *Two-Finger Technique (right photo):*
  a. Place the pads of two fingers on the infant's breastbone (sternum), with one touching and both below the imaginary nipple line.
  b. Give 30 chest compressions:
    • Push hard: about 1.5 inches (4 cm) straight down (at least one-third of the chest's diameter). If unable to the achieve the appropriate depth, use the heel of one hand instead of two fingers.
    • Push fast: to the beat of the Bee Gees song "Stayin' Alive".
    • At the end of each compression, let the infant's chest come back up to its normal position.

Skill Sheet 2-2 Infant CPR   *(Continued)*

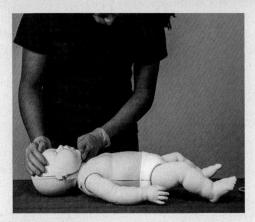

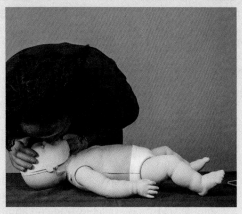

5 **A = Airway.**
Open the infant's airway using the head tilt–chin lift maneuver. **DO NOT** tilt the head back too far (less than for an adult or child).

6 **B = Breaths.**
a. Cover the infant's mouth with a mouth-to-barrier device if possible. If not possible, cover the infant's mouth and nose with your mouth and make an airtight seal. If this does not work, try either mouth-to-mouth or mouth-to-nose breaths.
b. Give 2 breaths, each lasting 1 second, to make the infant's chest rise.
c. Take a normal breath for yourself after each breath.
d. Continue CPR until one of the following occurs:
   • The infant begins breathing.
   • EMS arrives and takes over.
   • You become physically exhausted and are unable to continue.
e. If another person is available, trade off about every 5 sets of CPR (2 minutes).

Compression-Only CPR

Compression-only CPR, or hands-only CPR, is CPR without breaths. It intends to increase bystander involvement when CPR is needed for a person in cardiac arrest. Compression-only CPR is easy to teach, remember, and perform compared with conventional CPR. It may be used with adults or children, but not infants. (It is important to note that breaths are an important part of CPR with infants. Compression-only CPR in infants is *not* as effective as CPR with breaths. Compression-only CPR can even be detrimental for infants. Therefore, compression-only CPR should only be used with adults and children.)

A bystander who sees a person suddenly collapse and is not breathing but who is unable or unwilling to make mouth-to-mouth contact or unable to perform CPR can:

1. Ask another person to call 9-1-1 or an emergency response number.
2. Place the person face up on a flat, firm surface.
3. Push the center of the chest hard and fast (faster than 1 per second or use the beat of the Bee Gees song "Stayin' Alive"), the beats from a smartphone app that was previously installed and is quickly accessible, or a dispatcher's directions heard over a mobile phone's speaker.
4. Continue chest compressions without stopping until help arrives or as long as possible. If another person is available, trade off about every 2 minutes.

CPR Performance Mistakes

Mistakes made while performing CPR can usually be placed into one of the following two categories:

1. Rescue breathing mistakes:
   - Failing to ensure adequate head tilt-chin lift (airway will be closed)
   - Failing to pinch the nose shut in a child and adult or not covering mouth and nose in an infant
   - Failure to give slow breaths (lasting 1 second each)
   - Providing breaths that are too fast or too forceful
   - Failing to watch the person's chest rise and fall
   - Failing to maintain a tight seal around the mouth or barrier device
2. Chest compression mistakes:
   - Pivoting at knees instead of hips (eg, rocking motion)
   - Using the wrong compression site (eg, too high or too low on the chest)
   - Bending elbows (arms should be kept straight with elbows locked)
   - Failing to place shoulders above sternum (arms should be vertical)
   - Touching your fingers to the person's chest
   - Providing quick, stabbing compressions
   - Failing to allow the chest to fully recoil (eg, leaning on the chest)
   - Failing to keep your hand in contact with the person's chest between each compression (some instructors teach to lift hands off the chest, which allows the chest to recoil, but this could lead to stabbing compressions)

Recovery Position

If a person is unresponsive and breathing, place them in the side-lying recovery position (**FIGURE 2-1**). This position provides the following advantages:

- Helps keep the airway open.
- Allows fluids (eg, blood, vomit, mucus) to drain out of the nose and mouth and not into the throat.
- Allows the first aid responder, when alone, to leave to call for help.

Place the person (usually by rolling) on their side, using the following points:

- Bottom arm: Extend outward.
- Top arm: Rest arm on bicep of bottom arm.
- Top hand: Keep under the person's cheek to cushion it, keep the airway open, and allow fluids to drain.
- Top leg: Adjust so both the knee and hip are bent at right angles to serve as a prop.
- Head: Attempt to extend the chin while pointing the mouth downward.

If a neck, back, hip, or pelvic injury is suspected:

- DO NOT move the person. Leave the person in the position in which they were found.
- If the airway is blocked or the area is unsafe, move the person only as needed to open the airway or to reach a safe location. If moving them is necessary, support the head and neck while keeping the person's nose and navel pointing in the same direction.

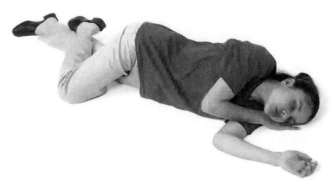

FIGURE 2-1 Recovery position.
© Jones & Bartlett Learning.

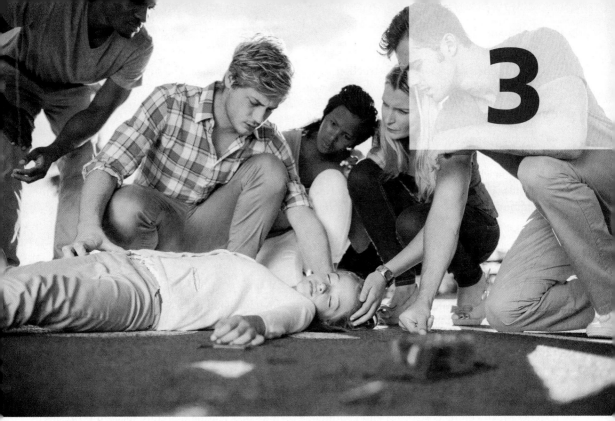

Airway Obstruction and Choking Care

Airway Obstruction

The human body requires a constant supply of oxygen from the air a person breathes. Breathing is the process of moving air in and out of the lungs. An object stuck in the throat's airway can affect breathing and be life threatening.

Recognizing Airway Obstruction

An object lodged in the airway can cause a mild or severe airway obstruction. In a mild airway obstruction, good air exchange is present and the person is able to make forceful coughing efforts in an attempt to relieve the obstruction. The person should be encouraged to cough.

A person with a severe airway obstruction will have poor air exchange. The signs of a severe airway obstruction include the following:

- Increased breathing difficulty
- Weak and ineffective cough
- Unable to speak or breathe
- Skin, fingernail beds, inside of mouth, or lips turn blue or gray

The person who is choking may also appear panicky and desperate and may hold their neck with one or both hands. This motion is known as the universal distress signal for choking. Another way a person might communicate that they are choking is by pointing a finger at their mouth.

Caring for Airway Obstruction

Adult and Child Airway Obstruction

The American Heart Association (AHA) recommends providing abdominal thrusts for dislodging an airway obstruction (choking) in a responsive adult or child older than 1 year. However, the International Liaison Committee on Resuscitation (ILCOR) recommends a combination of back blows and abdominal thrusts (5 back blows followed by 5 abdominal thrusts, known as the 5 and 5 approach) for airway obstruction.

Past editions of this book have not included back blows for dislodging an airway obstruction because AHA has not provided a recommendation on their use. However, back blows are recommended by ILCOR, which conducts rigorous and continuous reviews of scientific literature focused on resuscitation, cardiac arrest, and conditions requiring first aid. This organization's 2020 guidelines provide the justification for delivering back blows or a combination of back blows and abdominal thrusts for choking.

Some training organizations do not teach the back blow technique, only the abdominal thrust procedures. However, both approaches can be effective. An airway obstruction is a life-threatening event, so it is a good idea to know several procedures that can be used if others have failed.

If...	Then...
The person is responsive and shows signs of mild airway obstruction (choking): - Good air exchange is present - Able to make forceful coughing efforts in an attempt to relieve the obstruction	- Encourage continued coughing, but do nothing else. Aggressive treatment (eg, back blows, abdominal thrusts, chest compressions) may cause complications and could worsen the airway obstruction. - Monitor the person until they improve, because a severe airway obstruction can occur anytime.
The person is responsive and shows signs of complete airway obstruction: - Difficulty breathing - Unable to cough forcefully - Unable to talk - Skin, fingernail beds, or lips turn blue or gray - Appears panicky and desperate - Points to their mouth or grasps at their throat (**FIGURE 3-1**)	1. **DO NOT** ask them if they are okay. Instead, ask them if they are choking and if you can help them. If they nod "yes," tell them you are going to help. 2. Have someone call 9-1-1. 3. Stand to the side and slightly behind the choking person. 4. Support the person by placing one hand on the upper chest or shoulder or over the navel and have the person bend over at the waist to a 90° angle (their upper body should be parallel to the ground or floor). DO NOT keep them in an upright or vertical position. If they are not bending over when the jolt of the back blow dislodges the object, the object may become stuck deeper in the airway.

If...	Then...
Note: It is important to distinguish choking from fainting, heart attack, seizure, anaphylaxis, and other conditions that may cause sudden respiratory distress.	5. Give 5 hard back blows with the heel of the hand that is not supporting the person. Aim for the area in between their shoulder blades (**SKILL SHEET 3-1**). **DO NOT** just pat them on the back; use hard blows (eg, like driving or hitting a nail into a thick board with a hammer). 6. Check to see if each back blow has dislodged the obstruction. The aim is to relieve the object with a blow, not necessarily to give all 5 back blows or to give them as fast as possible. Each back blow should be a separate and distinct effort to dislodge the object.
The 5 back blows fail to dislodge the airway obstruction	1. Stand behind the person or kneel behind a child. If the person is a lot taller than you, have them kneel or sit. 2. Put one foot in front of the other foot; this provides stability during the thrusts and if the person becomes unresponsive and collapses, they can slide down your leg to the ground or floor. 3. Wrap your arms around the person's waist. Locate the person's navel (belly button) using two fingers (right-handed people will usually use their left hand). If your arms cannot encircle the person's waist (eg, pregnant woman, or a very large person and you are smaller than them), use chest thrusts. See below for chest thrust directions. 4. Make a fist with the other hand (right-handed people will usually use their right hand to make a fist). Place the thumb side of the fist just above the person's navel and below the tip of the breastbone (sternum). Grab the fist with the other hand. 5. Give up to 5 abdominal thrusts (**SKILL SHEET 3-2**) by quick inward and upward pulling of the fist into the person's abdomen. Each thrust should be a separate and distinct effort to dislodge the object, not to necessarily give all 5 abdominal thrusts.
The obstruction does not get dislodged and is still in place	Repeat alternating between back blows and abdominal thrusts until: • The person can cough forcefully, breathe, or speak, or • The person becomes unresponsive, or • EMS or someone with more advanced training takes over
The person becomes unresponsive or is found unresponsive	• Support the person while carefully lowering them to the ground. • If EMS have not arrived or have not been called, call them immediately. • Begin CPR, starting with chest compressions. Each time before giving the first of 2 breaths, open the mouth and look for an object.
Solid material or an object can be seen in the airway	Remove the solid material or object only if seen. **DO NOT** use a blind finger sweep.
The person is pregnant, very large, or if you are small	Provide chest thrusts (**FIGURE 3-2**): 1. Position yourself behind the person. 2. Put your arms under the person's armpits and your hands on the lower half of the breastbone (sternum). 3. Pull your hands straight back into the chest.
The object has been dislodged and the person has a persistent cough or feels something is stuck in their throat	Seek professional medical care because injuries may have occurred.

Skill Sheet 3-1 Adult or Child Choking: Back Blows

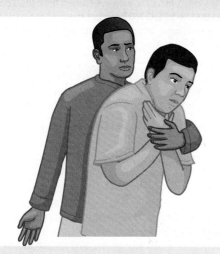

1 Stand behind the person and slightly to one side. Reach across the person's chest by wrapping one arm either over the person's arm or under their armpit. Place the palm of that hand on the person's upper chest or shoulder. Leave your other hand free.

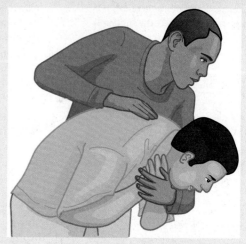

2 Have the person bend over at the waist to a 90° angle (their upper body should be parallel to the ground or floor). **DO NOT** keep them in an upright or a vertical position. If they are not bending over when the jolt of the back blow dislodges the object, the dislodged object may become stuck deeper in the airway.

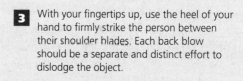

3 With your fingertips up, use the heel of your hand to firmly strike the person between their shoulder blades. Each back blow should be a separate and distinct effort to dislodge the object.

4 If 5 back blows do not dislodge the object, give up to 5 abdominal thrusts. (See Skill Sheet 3-2.)

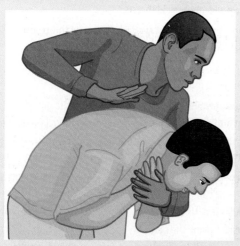

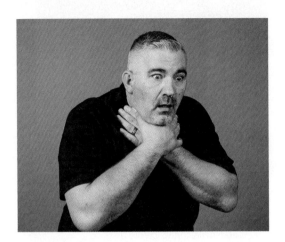

FIGURE 3-1 Universal sign for choking.
© Jones & Bartlett Learning.

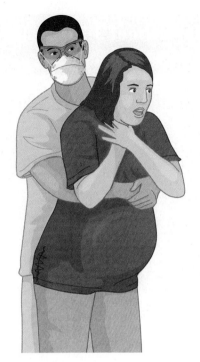

FIGURE 3-2 Chest thrusts are similar to CPR chest compressions, but are sharper and delivered at a slower rate. Hands are placed on the lower half of the breastbone (sternum).
© Jones & Bartlett Learning.

Skill Sheet 3-2 Adult or Child Choking: Abdominal Thrusts

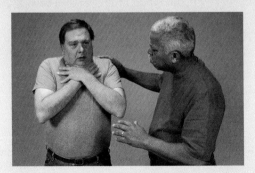

1 If the 5 back blows do not dislodge the object or the person is still unable to speak (see Skill Sheet 3-1), give up to 5 abdominal thrusts. Do this by following the remaining steps.

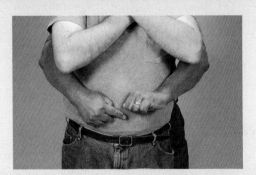

2 Stand behind an adult; stand or kneel behind a child. Wrap your arms around the person's waist. Locate the person's navel with a couple of fingers (right-handed people will usually use their left hand).

(Continues)

Skill Sheet 3-2 Adult or Child Choking: Abdominal Thrusts
(Continued)

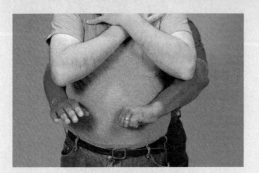 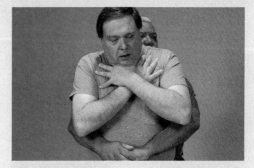

3 Make a fist with the other hand (right-handed people will usually use their right hand) and place the thumb side of that hand just above the person's navel and below the tip of the breastbone (sternum).

4 Grasp the fist with the other hand. Thrust the fist into the person's abdomen with a quick upward motion. Each thrust should be a separate and distinct effort to dislodge the object. After each thrust, quickly determine if the abdominal thrust dislodged the object. The aim is to relieve the object with a thrust, not to necessarily give all 5 abdominal thrusts before checking.

5 If the 5 abdominal thrusts do not dislodge the object, give up to 5 back blows again. Repeat a combination of 5 back blows and 5 abdominal thrusts until one of the following occurs:
- The object is dislodged and the person starts breathing.
- EMS or a person with more advanced training arrives and takes over.
- Another person arrives, allowing you to take turns giving back blows and abdominal thrusts.
- The person becomes unresponsive and collapses to the ground or floor.

6 If the person becomes unresponsive or a person is found unresponsive, then look in the mouth for an object. If seen, remove the object, then provide CPR by doing the following:
  a. Give 30 chest compressions.
  b. Give 2 breaths. If the first breath does not cause the chest to rise, retilt the head and attempt a second breath.
  c. Continue sets of 30 chest compressions and 2 breaths. Each time before giving the first of the 2 breaths, look into the mouth for an object; if seen, remove it.

© Jones & Bartlett Learning.

Infant Airway Obstruction

For a responsive infant with an airway obstruction, give back blows and chest thrusts instead of abdominal thrusts to relieve the obstruction:

1. Support the infant's head and neck and lay the infant facedown on your forearm, then lower your arm holding the infant onto your thigh.
2. Give 5 back blows between the infant's shoulder blades with the heel of your hand.

3. While supporting the back of the infant's head, roll the infant face up onto the other thigh and give 5 chest thrusts with 2 fingers on the infant's sternum in the same location used for CPR. These are separate and distinct thrusts and are not like the faster CPR compressions.
4. Repeat these steps until the object is removed or the infant becomes unresponsive.

For an infant with an airway obstruction, follow the steps in **SKILL SHEET 3-3**.

Skill Sheet 3-3 Infant Choking

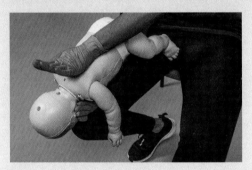
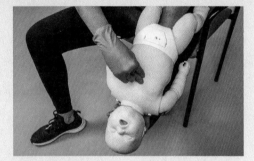

1 Give up to 5 separate and distinct back blows.
   a. Support the infant's head with your hand.
   b. Lay the infant facedown over your forearm, with the head lower than their chest.
   c. Brace your forearm and the infant against your thigh. (If holding the infant with your right hand and forearm, brace them against your right thigh; if using the left hand and arm, brace them against your left thigh.)
   d. Give 5 back blows between the infant's shoulder blades with the heel of your other hand.
   e. If the object does not come out, turn the infant onto their back while supporting the head.

2 Give up to 5 separate and distinct chest thrusts.
   a. Support the infant's head with your hand.
   b. Lay the infant faceup over your other forearm, tilt your arm down so the infant's head is lower than their chest.
   c. Brace your forearm and the infant against your other thigh.
   d. Place two fingers of your other hand in the same location as giving CPR compressions.
   e. Give the thrusts 1 second apart—this is not as fast as CPR compressions.

3 Continue alternating the 5 back blows and 5 chest thrusts without interruption until the infant stops responding or can breathe, cough, or cry, or until EMS or a person who is trained takes over.

4 If the infant is found or becomes unresponsive:
   a. Give 30 chest compressions.
   b. If the first breath does not cause the chest to rise, retilt the head and attempt a second breath. Continue sets of 30 chest compressions and 2 breaths. Each time before giving the first of 2 breaths, look into the infant's mouth for an object; if seen, remove it.

© Jones & Bartlett Learning.

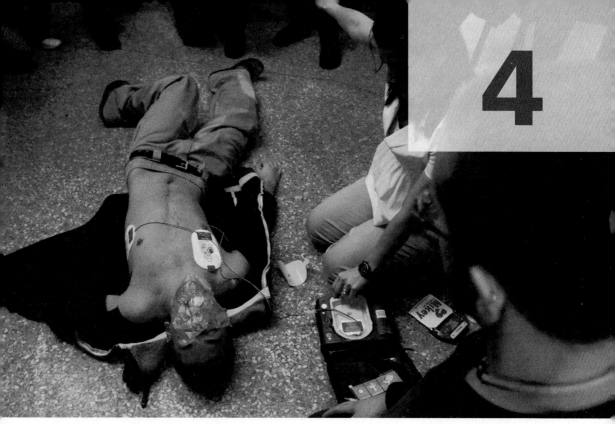

© Vince Talotta/Toronto Star/Getty Images.

Automated External Defibrillation

Automated External Defibrillators

More than 70% of all out-of-hospital cardiac arrests involve an irregular heart electrical rhythm or beat called ventricular fibrillation (VF). This condition involves the heart's ventricles (bottom two chambers of the heart) quivering or twitching and not producing effective heartbeats. In other words, no blood is pumped from the heart, and it is a form of cardiac arrest.

An automated external defibrillator (AED) analyzes the heart rhythm to determine if an electric shock, or defibrillation, is necessary. If it is, the AED will prompt the rescuer to deliver the shock to the heart of a person in cardiac arrest. The purpose of this shock is to correct an abnormal electrical disturbance and reestablish a heart rhythm that will result in normal electrical and pumping function. Using an AED as soon as possible increases the person's chance of survival.

The AED is attached to a cable that is connected to two adhesive pads (electrodes) that are placed on the person's chest. The pad and cable system send the electrical signal from the heart into the device for rhythm analysis and prompts the rescuer to deliver the electric shock to the person when needed. This system enables first aid responders and other rescuers to deliver early defibrillation with only minimal training.

Defibrillation is perhaps the single most effective therapeutic step for cardiac arrest.

Common Elements of AEDs

Many different AED models exist. The principles for use are the same for each, but the displays, controls, and options vary slightly. Do not let that intimidate you because most have voice prompts or visual displays to guide usage.

Using an AED

Once you have determined the need for the AED (person unresponsive and not breathing), the basic operation of all AED models follows the sequence in **SKILL SHEET 4-1**.

1. Some AEDs power on by pressing an on/off button. Others power on when the AED case lid is opened. Once the power is on, the AED will quickly go through some internal checks and will then begin to provide voice and/or screen prompts.
2. Expose the person's chest. The skin must be fairly dry so that the pads will adhere and conduct electricity properly. If necessary, dry the skin with a towel. Because excessive chest hair may also interfere with adhesion and electrical conduction, you may need to quickly shave the area where the pads are to be placed.
3. Remove the backing from the pads and apply them firmly to the person's bare chest according to the diagram on the pads. One pad is placed to the right of the breastbone, just below the collarbone and above the right nipple. The second pad is placed on the left side of the chest, left of the nipple and above the lower rib margin.
4. Make sure the cable is attached to the AED, and stand clear for analysis of the heart's electrical activity. No one should be in contact with the person at this time, or later if a shock is indicated.
5. Verify that no one is in contact with the person. The AED will advise you to push a button to administer the shock. Begin CPR immediately following the shock, and follow the prompts, which will include reanalyzing the heart rhythm (about every 5 sets of CPR [approximately 2 minutes]). If the shock worked, the person will begin to move. Assess the breathing and place the person into the recovery position to keep the airway clear. Continue providing care until EMS arrives and takes over.

DO NOT use the AED in water. Because water conducts electricity, the electrical current may move across the person's skin rather than between the pads to the person's heart. If the person is submerged in water, then pull them out of the water and quickly wipe off as much moisture as possible from the chest before attaching the AED pads.

Skill Sheet 4-1 Using an AED

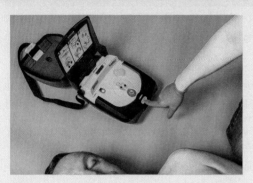

1 Turn on the AED.

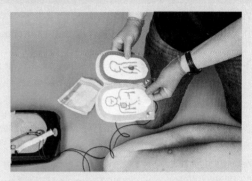

2 Attach the pads to the person's bare, dry chest (as shown on the pads). If needed, plug the cables into the AED.

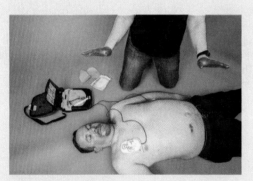

3 Stay clear of the person. Make sure no one, including yourself, is touching the person. Say, "Clear!"

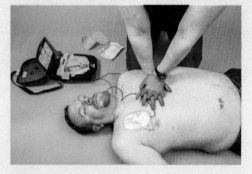

4 Allow the AED to analyze the heart. The AED will prompt one of two actions:
   a. Stay clear and press the shock button if advised to deliver a shock.
   b. Do not give shock but give CPR, starting with chest compressions with the pads staying in place.

5 After any one of the two actions, give 5 sets of CPR (approximately 2 minutes) unless the person moves, begins to breathe, or wakes up. Even if the person wakes up, leave AED pads on until EMS arrives.

6 Repeat Steps 3 and 4 until the person moves or begins to breathe, or until EMS takes over.

Special Considerations

What to Look For	What to Do
Wet skin, lying in shallow water, or on snow	• Move the person out of the water or off the snow. • Wipe the chest dry before attaching the pads.
Chest hair	Remove hair if it may prevent the pads from sticking to the skin. Do this by either: • Shaving the area where pads will be placed. The AED case should contain a razor to use, or • Apply adhesive tape (eg, duct, masking, bandage) firmly onto the hair and rip the tape off. It may be necessary to repeat this several times. If you have two or more sets of AED pads and adhesive tape is not available, you can use the AED pads to rip out hair. **DO NOT** use the AED pads to rip out hair if you only have one set of pads.
Medication patches (eg, nitroglycerin, nicotine, pain medication)	• While wearing gloves, or using a cloth or paper towel, remove the patch. • **DO NOT** place an AED pad over a medicine patch.
Implanted devices (pacemaker or defibrillator)	Move the pad at least 2 inches (5 cm) away from the device. **DO NOT** place an AED pad over the implanted device.
Child or infant	The procedure is the same as for an adult. Some AEDs may have pediatric AED pads. If the pads may touch each other, place one pad in the middle of the chest and the other pad on the back, between the shoulder blades. They should be separated by at least two finger widths (1 inch [2.5 cm]). If pediatric equipment is not available, use the adult equipment.

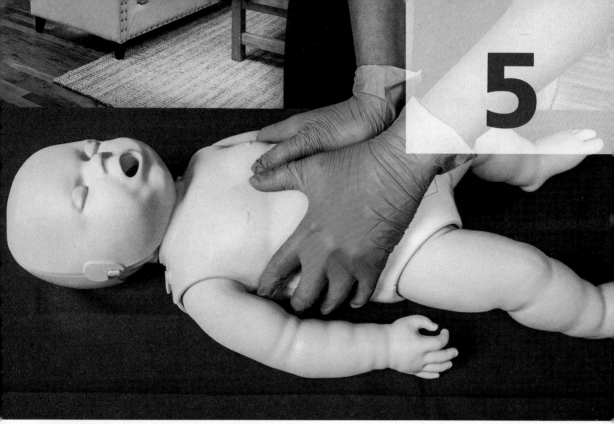

© Jones & Bartlett Learning.

CPR Precautions, Complications, and Special Situations

CPR Performance Mistakes

Mistakes made while performing cardiopulmonary resuscitation (CPR) can usually be placed into one of two categories:

1. Rescue breathing mistakes:
   - Failing to ensure adequate head tilt–chin lift (airway will be closed, **FIGURE 5-1**)
   - Failing to pinch the nose shut
   - Failing to give slow breaths (lasting 1 second each)
   - Providing breaths that are too fast or too forceful
   - Failing to watch the person's chest rise and fall
   - Failing to maintain a tight seal around the mouth or barrier device

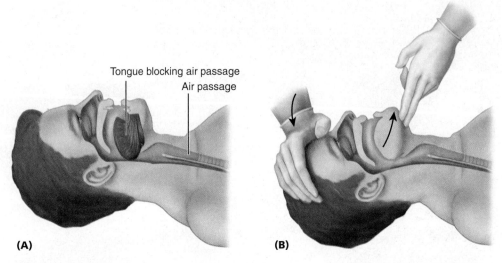

Tongue blocking air passage
Air passage

(A)   **(B)**

FIGURE 5-1 A. Relaxation of the tongue back into the throat causes airway obstruction. **B.** To perform the head tilt–chin lift maneuver, place one hand on the person's forehead and apply firm backward pressure with your palm to tilt the head back. Next, place the tips of the index and middle fingers of your other hand under the lower jaw near the bony part of the chin. Lift the chin upward, bringing the entire lower jaw with it, helping to tilt the head back.
© Jones & Bartlett Learning.

2. Chest compression mistakes:
   - Pivoting at knees instead of hips (ie, rocking motion)
   - Using the wrong compression site (ie, too high or too low on the chest)
   - Bending elbows (arms should be kept straight with elbows locked)
   - Failing to place shoulders above the sternum (arms should be vertical)
   - Touching your fingers to the person's chest
   - Providing quick, stabbing compressions
   - Failing to allow the chest to fully recoil (ie, leaning on the person's chest)
   - Failing to keep your hands in contact with the person's chest between each compression (some instructors teach to slightly lift hands off the chest, which allows the chest to recoil, but it could lead to stabbing compressions)
   - Failing to swap responders often enough and therefore becoming tired while providing CPR

Precautions During Training

- **DO NOT** practice mouth-to-mouth resuscitation on people; practice on a manikin.
- **DO NOT** practice chest compressions on people; practice on a manikin.
- **DO NOT** practice back blows, abdominal thrusts, or chest thrusts on people; practice on a specialized manikin for abdominal thrusts, if available.
- Wash your hands before and after class.
- Before using the manikin, clean it according to your instructor's directions. Use either a solution of liquid bleach and water or rubbing alcohol.
- **DO NOT** put anything (eg, chewing gum, food, drink, tobacco) in your mouth when manikins are being used.

Disease Precautions During CPR Training

Participants in CPR training are often concerned about getting diseases, such as acquired immunodeficiency syndrome (AIDS; from contracting the human immunodeficiency virus [HIV]), hepatitis (from contracting the hepatitis B virus), COVID-19, and respiratory tract infections (eg, influenza, mononucleosis, and tuberculosis) from a CPR manikin. CPR classes should follow the manikin manufacturers' recommendations for using and maintaining their manikins.

DO NOT use a training manikin if you have any of the following:

- Sores on the hands, lips, or face (eg, cold sore)
- An upper respiratory infection (eg, cold or sore throat)
- Hepatitis infection
- HIV or AIDS infection
- An infection or a recent exposure to an infectious source

Clean the manikin between each participant's use by doing the following:

1. Vigorously scrub the manikin's entire face and inside of the mouth with a 4×4 inch (10 ×10 cm) gauze pad that has been wet with 70% alcohol (eg, isopropanol or ethanol).
2. Place the wet gauze pad over the manikin's mouth and nose for at least 30 seconds.
3. Allow the manikin's face to dry.

Disease Precautions During Actual CPR

Mouth-to-Barrier Devices

Laypeople are most likely to perform CPR in the home (70% of the time) and will usually know the health status of the person. However, people may be unwilling to help a person in need because they fear contracting a disease. They should learn how to use a mouth-to-barrier device (eg, pocket mask or face shield).

Two types of mouth-to-barrier devices exist (**FIGURE 5-2**):

1. *Pocket masks.* These have a one-way valve so that exhaled air does not enter the responder's mouth. Devices without one-way valves offer little protection.
2. *Face shields.* These have no exhalation valve, and air can leak around the shield.

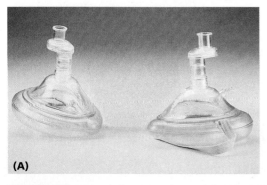
(A)

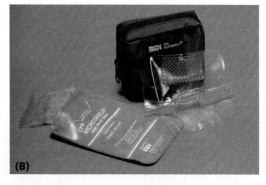
(B)

FIGURE 5-2 Barrier devices. **A.** Pocket mask for CPR. **B.** Face shields for CPR.
A. © Jones & Bartlett Learning. Courtesy of MIEMSS; B. © Jones & Bartlett Learning.

If a responder refuses to give rescue breaths, they should activate the emergency medical services (EMS) system and give chest compressions until a responder arrives who will give rescue breaths.

Other Personal Protective Equipment

Lay responders should avoid contact with blood and other body fluids by putting on personal protective equipment (PPE). PPE includes disposable medical exam gloves, eye protection, and, if providing compression-only CPR, face coverings for public health such as a face mask or shield to prevent disease transmission. (See pages 7–8.)

When NOT to Start CPR

Although CPR usually should be started whenever a person is not breathing, there are situations in which CPR should not be attempted. **DO NOT** start CPR in the following situations:

- The provision of CPR will place you at risk of serious injury or infectious disease.
- Signs of death are present:
  - Severe mutilation or decapitation
  - Rigor mortis (stiffening of muscles and body rigidity that starts developing 1 to 2 hours after death)
  - Evidence of tissue decomposition
  - Lividity (body parts closest to the ground have a purple-red appearance)
- The person has been in cardiac arrest for more than 30 minutes without receiving resuscitation efforts. Exceptions include situations involving drowning and hypothermia.
- The person has a do-not-resuscitate (DNR) order (usually in writing and decided on by the person's family and physician).

Dangerous Complications

Suspected Spinal Injury

To open the airway in persons with a suspected spinal injury, first aid responders should initially use manual spinal motion restriction (eg, placing their hands on the sides of the person's head to hold it still). **DO NOT** apply a cervical collar. Use of a cervical collar by lay first aid responders may be harmful.

Vomiting

Vomiting may occur during CPR. If it happens, it is usually before CPR has begun or within the first minute after beginning CPR. If the person receiving CPR inhales vomit (aspiration) into the lungs, a type of pneumonia can result that can kill the person even after successful rescue efforts.

In the event of vomiting, do the following:

1. Turn the person onto their side and keep them there until vomiting ends.
2. To clear the airway, wipe vomit out of the person's mouth with your fingers wrapped in a cloth or gauze or while wearing disposable gloves.
3. Reposition the person onto their back and resume CPR if needed.

Stomach Distention

Stomach (gastric) distention describes a stomach that is bulging from air. This condition is especially common in children and is caused by the following:

- Rescue breaths given too fast
- Rescue breaths given too forcefully
- Partially or completely blocked airway

Stomach distention is dangerous because the air in the stomach pushes against the lungs, making it difficult or impossible for responders to give full breaths. It also increases the possibility of the person inhaling vomit into the lungs. To prevent or minimize the risk of this condition, do the following:

1. Try to blow just hard enough to make the chest rise.
2. Retilt the head to open the airway.
3. Provide slow rescue breaths, pausing between breaths to take another breath.
4. **DO NOT** try to push air out of the stomach. Retilt the person's head and continue providing breaths for 1 second. If the person vomits, turn the person onto their side. To clear the airway, wipe vomit out of the person's mouth with your fingers wrapped in a cloth or gauze or while wearing disposable gloves. Roll the person onto their back, and continue CPR.

Inhalation of Foreign Substances

Inhalation of foreign substances (known as aspiration) can occur before or during rescue efforts (CPR or abdominal thrusts). There are three types of foreign substances that may be aspirated:

- Particulate matter (can obstruct an airway)
- Nongastric liquid (mainly related to drowning)
- Gastric acid (the effects of gastric acid aspiration on lung tissue can be equated with a chemical burn)

If an unresponsive person vomits, roll the person onto one side and wipe the mouth clean. To clear the person's airway, wipe vomit out of their mouth with your fingers wrapped in a cloth or gauze or while wearing disposable gloves. Afterward, continue providing care.

Chest Compression–Related Injuries

Chest compression–related injuries can happen even with proper compression technique. Injuries may include rib fractures or separation, a bruised lung, or lung or liver lacerations. To prevent or minimize the risk of chest compression–related injuries, do the following:

1. Properly locate your hands on the person's chest (**FIGURE 5-3**). If your hands are too low, the tip of the person's sternum can cut or injure the liver.
2. Keep your fingers off of the person's ribs by interlocking your fingers and using the heel of your hand on the chest.
3. Press straight down instead of sideways.
4. Give smooth, regular, and uninterrupted compressions (except when giving rescue breaths).
5. Avoid pressing the chest too deeply.

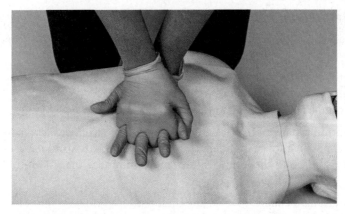

FIGURE 5-3 The proper hand position for chest compressions is in the center of the chest.
© Jones & Bartlett Learning.

Dentures, Loose or Broken Teeth, or Dental Appliances

Leave tight-fitting dentures in place to make a better seal for rescue breathing. Remove loose or broken teeth, dentures, and/or dental appliances, which may fall back into the person's throat and the airway.

Special Resuscitation Situations

The following conditions have been identified in recent CPR guidelines as special resuscitation situations involving CPR.

Care for a Person Experiencing a Stroke

Stroke is caused by a blockage (**FIGURE 5-4**) or rupture of a blood vessel in the brain (**FIGURE 5-5**) that prevents part of the brain from getting the blood flow it needs. The acronym FAST acts as an assessment tool to determine if a stroke may have occurred:

F = Face. Ask the person to smile. It is abnormal if one side of the face does not move well compared with the other side.

A = Arms. Ask the person to close their eyes and raise both arms with the palms up. It is abnormal if one arm drifts downward when held extended.

S = Speech. Ask the person to repeat a simple phrase (eg, "The sky is blue."). It is abnormal if the person slurs words, uses the wrong words, or cannot speak at all.

T = Time. Seek medical help if any of the preceding signs occur. The presence of one of these signs is associated with a high risk of stroke (72%); if all three are present, the risk is as high as 85%.

Call 9-1-1, and while waiting for EMS:

If...	Then...
The person is unresponsive and not breathing	Begin CPR.
The person is unresponsive and breathing	Place the person on their side in the recovery position. (See page 21.)

If...	Then...
If the person is breathing and alert	<ul><li>Position the person of their back with head and shoulders slightly raised.</li><li>Loosen tight or constricting clothing.</li><li>Be prepared to turn the person onto their side and into the recovery position to allow drool or vomit to drain.</li></ul>

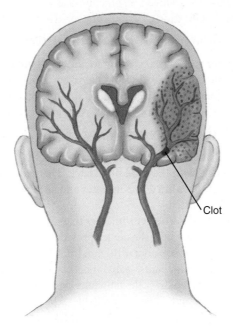

FIGURE 5-4 Blockage of a blood vessel in the brain.
© Jones & Bartlett Learning.

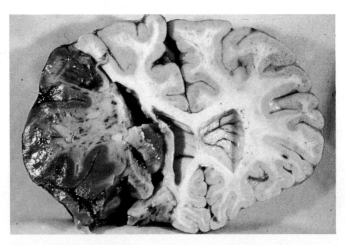

FIGURE 5-5 Rupture of a blood vessel in the brain.
© American Academy of Orthopaedic Surgeons.

CPR for a Person Experiencing an Opioid Overdose

Opioids are a classification of drugs that relieve pain. Opioids slow or even stop breathing. Drug overdoses can be fatal. In recent years, opioid-associated deaths have soared to tens of thousands per year.

A drug overdose can happen when a person:

- Misunderstands the directions for use, unintentionally takes an extra dose, or deliberately misuses a prescription opioid or an illicit drug (eg, heroin)
- Takes an opioid medication prescribed for someone else
- Mixes opioids with other medications, alcohol, or over-the-counter (OTC) drugs.

When an unresponsive person is known or suspected to have taken an opioid, check for breathing:

- If the person is not breathing or is only gasping for air and there is someone to help, have the other person call 9-1-1 and obtain an AED and naloxone, while you begin CPR.
- If the person is not breathing or is only gasping for air and you are alone, complete 5 cycles of CPR before leaving to call 9-1-1 and obtaining an AED and naloxone.

Then, give naloxone, if available (**FIGURE 5-6**).

- To administer a prefilled, single-dose nasal spray that cannot be reused (eg, Narcan), first place the person flat on their back, with the head tilted back. Then administer the spray into one nostril. If there is no recovery within 2 to 3 minutes and another nasal spray device is available, repeat the dose in the other nostril.
- To administer a prefilled, single-dose auto-injector that cannot be reused (eg, Evzio), pull the device out of the case. Once activated, the device provides voice directions (similar to automated defibrillators). Inject into the person's outer thigh (similar to an epinephrine auto-injector). It can be given through clothing (eg, pants, jeans) if necessary. If the electronic voice directions do not work, the device can still deliver the naloxone dose. If there is no recovery within 2 to 3 minutes and there is another auto-injector available, repeat the dose.
- If the person is still not breathing, continue CPR until EMS arrives.

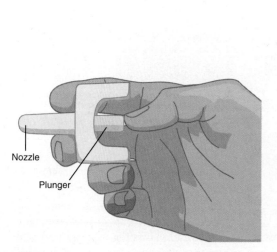
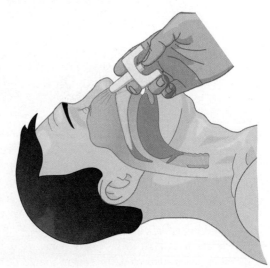

Nozzle

Plunger

FIGURE 5-6 Nasal spray naloxone administration.

CPR for a Person With Hypothermia

The person with severe hypothermia must be handled very gently. The cold heart is very prone to spontaneous ventricular fibrillation due to any movement. Even cautious movement of the person may induce ventricular fibrillation.

It is difficult to assess breathing in an unresponsive person with hypothermia. If the person is unresponsive and not breathing, check the person's heart rate for 1 minute (Check pulse on the neck's carotid artery on the side nearest you. Lay rescuers usually are not taught to check the carotid artery.) and then begin CPR. **DO NOT** wait to check the person's temperature, and **DO NOT** wait until the person is rewarmed to start CPR. Prevent further heat loss by removing the person's wet clothes; insulate and shield the person from wind and additional cold exposure. Avoid rough handling and activate the EMS system as soon as possible. Continue CPR until EMS arrives. In a person with severe hypothermia, CPR can be given intermittently during evacuation if it is not possible or safe to perform continuous CPR. CPR can be given for several hours, if necessary. Deliver chest compressions at 100 to 120 beats per minute.

DO NOT start CPR in the following situations:

- The person has been submerged in cold water for more than 1 hour.
- The person has obvious fatal injuries.
- The person is frozen (eg, ice in airway).
- The person's chest is stiff or compressions are not possible.
- Rescuers are exhausted or in danger.

CPR for a Person in an Avalanche

Avalanche-related deaths are on the rise in North America due to winter recreational activities (eg, backcountry skiing and snowboarding, helicopter and snowcat skiing, snowmobiling, out-of-bounds skiing, ice climbing, mountaineering, snowshoeing). The most common causes of avalanche-related death are suffocation (hypoxia), traumatic injury, hypothermia, or a combination of these factors. After the person has been uncovered and, if the person is unresponsive and is not breathing, begin CPR. Use an automated external defibrillator (AED) as soon as it becomes available. **DO NOT** attempt resuscitation in a person buried for 35 minutes or longer with an airway that is obstructed by snow or ice.

CPR for a Drowning Person

Give CPR as soon as an unresponsive submersed person is removed from the water. If you are alone, give 5 sets (about 2 minutes) of CPR before leaving the person to activate the EMS system and obtain an AED. If you are not alone, send someone to activate the EMS system and obtain an AED while you continue giving CPR. An AED should be used as soon as it becomes available.

People with only respiratory arrest usually respond after a few rescue breaths. Rescue breathing can be started once the person is in shallow water; however, chest compressions are difficult to perform in water and may not be effective. There is no need to attempt to clear the airway of water because only a small amount of water is aspirated by most drowning people and is absorbed by the body. **DO NOT** try to remove water by performing abdominal thrusts.

If vomiting occurs during CPR, turn the person onto their side. To clear the airway, wipe vomit out of the person's mouth with your fingers wrapped in a cloth or gauze or while wearing disposable gloves. If a spinal injury is suspected, the person should be turned as a unit with no twisting. A suggestion is to keep the person's nose and navel pointed in the same direction that they are being turned. Stop CPR after 30 minutes unless the person has hypothermia.

CPR for a Person Struck by Lightning

The National Weather Service estimates that an average of 49 deaths occur from lightning strikes in the United States each year (**FIGURE 5-7**). The main cause of death in these people is cardiac arrest. When multiple people are struck at the same time by lightning, rescuers should give the highest priority to people who are unresponsive and not breathing by beginning CPR. People struck by lightning are not electrically charged and can be touched. An AED should be used as soon as it becomes available.

CPR for a Person Infected With COVID-19

COVID-19 is an illness caused by a virus that can spread from person to person. A person can become infected from respiratory droplets when an infected person coughs, sneezes, or speaks. It may also be spread by touching a surface or object that has the virus on it, and then by touching your mouth, nose, eyes, or face, however this risk is considered to be low. Everyone is at risk of getting COVID-19. In addition to the COVID-19 pandemic, other respiratory-related epidemics and pandemics have and will continue in the future.

This presents a dilemma for a first aid responder who is concerned about compromising their own health and perhaps life, yet wants to give CPR as an attempt to save the life of a COVID-19 victim in cardiac arrest. If a person known to be infected with the COVID-19 virus is in cardiac arrest, perform compression-only CPR as described previously, with the addition of covering the person's nose and mouth with a cloth or face mask and the first aid responder wearing a mask to cover their own nose and mouth.

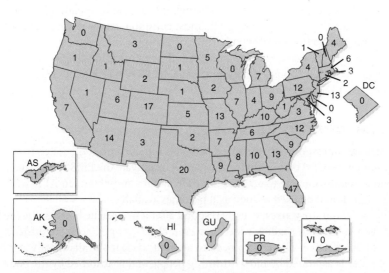

FIGURE 5-7 Lightning fatalities by state, 2007-2016.
Data from National Weather Service, compiled by Vaisala, Inc.

CPR for a Person With a Do-Not-Resuscitate Order

A lay responder cannot get into any legal trouble for giving CPR or other life saving treatment to a person with a do-not-resuscitate (DNR) order, and should always give such care as soon as possible to all persons and especially those experiencing a sudden cardiac arrest.

Good Samaritan laws in most states protect lay responders from legal consequences if they act prudently and adhere to their training.

Professional healthcare responders who give CPR or other life saving treatment to people with a DNR order as an attempt to save a life can potentially be in trouble—if they know about the DNR.

Laws and regulations vary by country, state, and locality. Therefore, it is advised that if you know someone with a DNR order to consult with the issuing physician or an attorney for applicable legal advice.

Appendix: CPR and AED Review

Using TABLE A-1, review CPR and AED procedures using the **RAB-CAB** sequence.

TABLE A-1 Quick Review of CPR and AED Procedures Using the RAB-CAB Sequence

Steps/action	Adults (at or past puberty)	Child (1 year to puberty)	Infant (younger than 1 year)
R = Responsive?			
Technique	Tap a shoulder and shout, "Are you OK?" A person or child who is responsive will answer, move, or moan.		Tap the bottom of a foot and shout their name. A responsive infant will cry or move.
A = Activate EMS and obtain an AED. **(Shout for nearby help and call 9-1-1 or the emergency response number. An AED may or may not be available.)**			
When?	■ If you are alone, call 9-1-1 and obtain an AED. When you return, use the AED. ■ If another person is with you, send them to call and obtain an AED while you begin CPR immediately.	■ If you are alone, and before calling 9-1-1, give 5 sets of 30 chest compressions and 2 breaths (CPR). ■ After 5 sets of CPR, call 9-1-1 and obtain an AED. ■ When you return, use the AED as soon as possible.	
Whom to call?	Call 9-1-1 or the emergency response number.		
B = Breathing? **(Check for no breathing or only gasping.)**			
■ Place person face-up on a flat, firm surface. ■ Observe from the neck to the waist movement for breathing. Take 5 seconds but no more than 10 seconds.	If the person is not breathing or is only occasionally gasping (may sound like a quick inhalation or like a groan/snore), CPR is needed. If the person is breathing but not responding, CPR is not needed; place the person in the recovery position to keep their airway clear, and monitor breathing.		
C = Chest compressions			
Where to place person?	Firm, flat surface (eg, floor, ground, sidewalk)		Can be placed on table or cabinet top

(Continues)

TABLE A-1 Quick Review of CPR and AED Procedures Using the RAB-CAB Sequence *(Continued)*

Steps/action	Adults (at or past puberty)	Child (1 year to puberty)	Infant (younger than 1 year)
Where to place hands?	Center of chest and lower half of breastbone (sternum)		Use one of the following techniques: ■ Encircling thumbs technique: Both thumbs on lower third of the breastbone, both touching the imaginary nipple line and the fingers encircling around the infant's back and chest ■ Two-finger technique: Pads of two fingers in the center of the chest on the breastbone with one finger touching and both below the imaginary nipple line
	Two hands: ■ Heel of one hand on breastbone; other hand on top ■ Fingers of both hands interlocked ■ Arms straight with shoulders directly over the hands	One hand for very small child: Heel of one hand only Two hands: ■ Same as for an adult ■ Arms straight with shoulders directly over the hands	
Depth	At least 2 inches (5 cm) but no more than 2.4 inches (6 cm)	About 2 inches (5 cm) or one-third depth of the upper body (chest)	About 1.5 inches (4 cm) or one-third depth of the upper body (chest)
	After each compression, allow full recoil of the chest. **DO NOT** lean on the chest of an adult or child.		
Rate	100 to 120 per minute (Follow the beat of the Bee Gees' song "Stayin' Alive", the beats from a smartphone application that was previously installed and is quickly accessible, or a dispatcher's directions heard over a cell phone's speaker.)		
Ratio of chest compressions to breaths	30:2		
A = Airway open			
Technique	Head tilt–chin lift maneuver		

TABLE A-1 Quick Review of CPR and AED Procedures Using the RAB-CAB Sequence *(Continued)*

Steps/action	Adults (at or past puberty)	Child (1 year to puberty)	Infant (younger than 1 year)
B = Breaths			

Technique	■ When possible, use a mouth-to-barrier device. If not possible, pinch the nose shut, and, with your mouth, make an airtight mouth-to-mouth seal. Use a CPR mask or face shield, if available.
	■ Perform the head tilt–chin lift maneuver.
	■ Give 2 breaths:
	  • Each breath should last 1 second.
	  • Blow enough to make the chest rise.
	If first breath does not cause chest to rise, retilt head and give second breath. If second breath does not make chest rise, begin CPR (30 compressions and 2 breaths). Each time before giving a breath, open the mouth and look for an object; if seen, remove it.
			Perform the head tilt–chin lift maneuver (do not tilt the head back too far).
			■ Cover the infant's mouth and nose with your mouth, making an airtight seal. If this does not work, try either mouth-to-mouth or mouth-to-nose breaths.
			■ Give 2 breaths:
			  • Each breath should last 1 second.
			  • Blow enough to make the chest rise.

Continue CPR until:

1. The person begins breathing.
2. Other rescuer(s) (eg, trained layperson, EMS personnel) take over.
3. An AED arrives and is used.
4. You become physically exhausted and unable to continue. (This might be prevented by having another person, if available, trade off every 5 sets of CPR [2 minutes]. Also, if the first aid responder is alone, they could consider performing compression-only CPR.)

Defibrillation

If available, use an AED as soon as possible. If another person is present, continue CPR while the other person prepares for AED use, or have that person continue CPR while you prepare for AED use.

1. Turn on the AED.
2. Attach the pads on the person's bare, dry chest (shown on the pads' diagrams). If needed, plug the cables into the AED. Child-sized pads may be available.
3. If you or another person is giving CPR, stop and stay clear of the person. Make sure no one, including you, is touching the person. Say, "Clear!"
4. Allow the AED to analyze the heart rhythm. The AED will prompt one of two actions:
   • Stay clear and press the shock button.
   • Do not shock but give CPR, starting with chest compressions with the pads staying in place.

After performing any one of the actions, give 5 sets of CPR (2 minutes) unless the person moves, begins to breathe, or wakes up. Even if the person wakes up, leave AED pads on until EMS arrives.

Repeat defibrillation Steps 3 and 4 until the person moves, begins to breathe, or wakes up, or EMS arrives and takes over.

Index

Note: Page numbers followed by *f* and *t* indicate figures and tables, respectively.